VITALITY CHRONICLES

Vol. 2

KNEE PAIN RELIEF EXERCISES FOR SENIORS

DR. ALEX WELLSPRING

All rights reserved.

No part of this publication may be reproduced, distributed, or transmitted in any form or by any means, including photocopying, recording, or other electronic or mechanical methods, without the prior written permission of the publisher, except in the case of brief quotations embodied in critical reviews and certain other noncommercial uses permitted by copyright law.

Copyright © Dr. Alex Wellspring, 2024.

TABLE OF CONTENTS

INTRODUCTION 6
CHAPTER 1: UNDERSTANDING KNEE PAIN 10
   Common Causes Of Knee Pain In Seniors 10
   Overview Of How Aging Affects The Knees 16
   Important Of Exercise For Treating Knee Discomfort 21
CHAPTER 2: BENEFITS OF EXERCISE FOR SENIORS 24
   Discussion On The Multiple Advantages Of Regular Exercise For Seniors 24
   How Exercise Can Help Relieve Knee Pain And Improve Mobility 27
   Introduction To The Concept Of Functional Fitness 30
      Key Elements of Functional Fitness 31
      The Benefits Of Functional Fitness 33
CHAPTER 3: SAFETY CONSIDERATIONS 36
   Tips For Safe Exercise As A Senior With Knee Pain 36
   The Need For Proper Warm-Up And Cool-Down Routines 40
      Warm-Up: Readying the Body for Action 40
      Cool-Down: Aiding Recovery and Relaxation 41
   Guidelines For Listening To Your Body And Avoiding Overexertion 44

CHAPTER 4: RANGE OF MOTION EXERCISES 48

Gentle Exercises To Enhance Flexibility And Range Of Motion In The Knees 48

The Significance Of Retaining Joint Mobility For Pain Alleviation 52

CHAPTER 5: STRENGTHENING EXERCISES 56

Introduction To Strength Training Routines That Are Especially Good For Seniors With Knee Pain 56

Important Considerations for Strength Training 58

Tips To Gradually Increase Resistance And Intensity 61

CHAPTER 6: BALANCE AND STABILITY TRAINING 64

The Significance Of Balance And Stability Exercises In Reducing Falls And Enhancing Knee Function 64

Demonstrations Of Exercises To Enhance Balance, Proprioception, And Coordination 67

    Exercise Demonstrations 67

Integrating Balancing Issues Into Regular Activities 71

CHAPTER 7: LOW-IMPACT CARDIOVASCULAR EXERCISES 74

Overview Of The Advantages Of Cardiovascular Exercise For Knee Health 74

Introduction To Low-Impact Exercises For Seniors With Knee Pain 78

Tips To Maintain Cardiovascular Fitness Without Exacerbating Knee Issues 81

CHAPTER 8: MIND-BODY EXERCISES 84

Investigation Of Mind-Body Methods For Controlling Knee Pain 84

- Practicing Yoga To Reduce Knee Pain 85
- Demonstrating Yoga for Knee Pain Relief 85
- Tai Chi For Knee Pain Relief 88
- Meditation and Deep Breathing Exercises 88

Mind-Body Activities May Improve General Well-Being 90

CHAPTER 9: LIFESTYLE MODIFICATIONS 96

Tips For Changing Your Lifestyle To Improve Knee Health And Pain Management 96

Guidelines For Maintaining A Healthy Weight, Good Eating, And Enough Water 99

Proper Footwear And Ergonomics Are Important For Preventing Knee Discomfort 103

- Proper Footwear 103
- Ergonomics 105

CHAPTER 10: LONG-TERM MAINTENANCE AND SUPPORT 108

Strategies For Sustaining Improvement And Avoiding Recurrence Of Knee Pain 108

Resources For Continued Assistance And Advice *111*
CONCLUSION 114

INTRODUCTION

Welcome to **Vitality Chronicles Vol. 2.** In this book, we'll go on a trip to uncover effective ways to manage knee pain and improve overall quality of life. Whether you are a senior suffering knee discomfort or someone looking to assist a loved one on their quest for improved knee health, this book will give you helpful ideas and practical activities to aid you on your way to wellness.

Knee pain is a typical problem for many seniors, and it may be caused by several reasons including arthritis, accidents, and ordinary wear and tear. This discomfort may have a substantial influence on everyday living, making basic actions like walking, climbing stairs, and even standing difficult and uncomfortable. However, with the appropriate technique, it is possible to relieve the pain while regaining mobility and independence.

One of the book's main advantages is its emphasis on exercise as a method of reducing knee discomfort. Exercise is an effective technique for improving strength, flexibility, and balance, all of which are necessary for supporting the knees and lowering discomfort. Through a series of mild exercises and stretches, you will learn how to strengthen the muscles surrounding the knees, increase flexibility, and decrease stiffness, resulting in reduced discomfort and better mobility.

But this book contains more than simply exercises. It also discusses the necessity of lifestyle changes and adequate self-care practices in controlling knee discomfort. From adequate diet and hydration guidelines to advise on keeping a healthy weight and integrating relaxation methods into your daily routine, this book offers a comprehensive approach to knee pain treatment that covers both the physical and emotional elements of the condition.

The influence on individuals who bought this book and put its techniques into action has been remarkable. Many people have experienced great pain relief, improved mobility, and a revived feeling of independence and well-being. Readers who followed the exercises and guidance described in this book were able to regain control of their knee health and enhance their general quality of life.

As you begin your journey through this book, I urge you to approach it with an open mind and a dedication to your health and well-being. Each chapter builds on the previous one, bringing you through a series of exercises and lifestyle modifications that will allow you to take control of your knee health and live a more active, pain-free life.

So, prepare to plunge in, learn, develop, and heal. These sections provide all of the information and resources you will need to optimize your knee health. By the conclusion of this book, you'll have the healing and knowledge you need to live your life to the fullest.

CHAPTER 1: UNDERSTANDING KNEE PAIN

Common Causes Of Knee Pain In Seniors

Knee discomfort is a common problem among seniors, frequently affecting their quality of life and mobility. As people age, their knees experience natural wear and tear, rendering them vulnerable to a variety of ailments and injuries. Understanding the most frequent causes of knee pain in seniors is critical for developing effective treatment and preventative methods.

1. **Osteoarthritis (OA):** Osteoarthritis is a common cause of knee discomfort in the elderly. It is a degenerative joint disease marked by the progressive disintegration of cartilage, the protective tissue that cushions the ends of bones in the joint. As cartilage deteriorates, bones may rub together, resulting in discomfort, stiffness, and inflammation. Seniors with osteoarthritis often feel increasing discomfort during movement or weight-bearing activities like walking or climbing stairs. Age, genetics, obesity, and past joint traumas all raise the chance of getting OA.

2. **Rheumatoid Arthritis (RA):** Rheumatoid arthritis is an autoimmune condition that affects individuals of all ages, although its frequency rises with age, especially among seniors. RA attacks the synovium, the lining of the joint capsule, as opposed to osteoarthritis, which largely affects the cartilage. Chronic inflammation in the synovium may destroy cartilage and bone, causing knee discomfort, edema, and stiffness. Seniors with RA may also have systemic symptoms including weariness and fever. Early diagnosis and treatments are critical for controlling RA and reducing its effect on knee health.

3. **Degenerative Meniscus Tears:** The meniscus is a C-shaped cartilage structure that functions as a stress absorber in the knee joint. The meniscus may degrade with age or repeated stress, making it more prone to tears. Seniors with degenerative meniscus tears may suffer knee discomfort, swelling, and locking or catching sensations, especially during twisting or pivoting. While acute meniscus tears are prevalent in young people as a result of sporting injuries, degenerative tears are more common in older persons and may need conservative therapy or surgical intervention, depending on their severity.

4. **Patellofemoral Pain Syndrome (PFPS):** Patellofemoral pain syndrome, often known as runner's knee, is a prevalent cause of knee discomfort in seniors, particularly those who

participate in activities that require repeated knee bending, such as walking, squatting, or ascending stairs. PFPS causes discomfort around or below the kneecap (patella), which might aggravate with extended sitting, kneeling, or descending stairs. Weak quadriceps muscles, incorrect kneecap alignment, and changes in joint mechanics caused by osteoarthritis or muscle imbalances are all factors that contribute to PFPS in seniors.

5. **Bursitis:** Bursae are tiny fluid-filled sacs that surround the knee joint and serve to decrease tissue friction. Bursitis develops when these sacs become inflamed owing to repeated stress, trauma, or underlying disorders like osteoarthritis. Seniors suffering from knee bursitis may have localized discomfort, swelling, and soreness, notably around the bony protrusion on the front of the knee (prepatellar bursitis) or the inside side of the knee (pes anserine bursitis). Rest, ice therapy, anti-inflammatory medicines, and physical therapy are common treatments used to ease symptoms and prevent recurrence.

6. **Traumatic Injury:** While age-related deterioration is the most common cause of knee discomfort in seniors, traumatic injuries including fractures, ligament tears, and tendon ruptures may also occur, particularly after falls or accidents. Patellar or proximal tibial fractures are more likely in elderly persons with weakening bones (osteoporosis). Ligament injuries, such as anterior cruciate ligament (ACL) rupture,

may happen during activities that require rapid pauses or changes in direction. Prompt medical examination and treatment are critical for improving results and avoiding long-term consequences.

7. **Gout:** Gout is a kind of arthritis characterized by the buildup of urate crystals in the joints, causing abrupt and intense bouts of pain, swelling, and redness. Gout may affect any joint, however, it usually affects the big toe, ankle, or knee. Seniors with gout may endure occasional flare-ups caused by dietary variables, alcohol intake, or certain medicines. Long-term gout care includes lifestyle adjustments, dietary changes, and drugs to decrease uric acid levels and minimize flare-ups.

8. **Post-Traumatic Arthritis:** Post-traumatic arthritis may occur in seniors who have previously had knee injuries, such as fractures or ligament tears, that impair the joint's natural mechanics. Over time, damaged joint surfaces may cause faster wear and tear, culminating in arthritis. Seniors with post-traumatic arthritis may have growing joint pain, stiffness, and edema for years after the original incident. Depending on the level of joint injury, treatment options may range from conservative methods such as physical therapy and pain management to surgical techniques such as joint replacement.

9. **Obesity:** Excess body weight is a major risk factor for knee discomfort and osteoarthritis in seniors. Obesity puts extra strain on the knee joints, hastening the degenerative process and increasing the risk of experiencing knee discomfort. Seniors who are overweight or obese may benefit from weight reduction measures, such as diet and exercise, to lessen the strain on their knees and improve overall joint health. Even little weight reduction may result in considerable pain and function benefits in people with knee osteoarthritis.

10. **The Lifestyle Factors:** Certain lifestyle factors might lead to knee discomfort in older adults. Prolonged periods of inactivity or sedentary behavior may cause muscular weakening and joint stiffness, worsening knee discomfort. In contrast, participating in high-impact activities or using inappropriate training methods might raise the risk of knee injury and hasten joint degradation. Seniors are advised to be active, with an emphasis on low-impact activities that improve joint mobility, muscular strength, and cardiovascular health.

To summarize, knee pain is a common and frequently debilitating condition for seniors, with a variety of variables contributing to its development and progression. Understanding the most frequent causes of knee pain in older individuals allows healthcare practitioners to personalize treatment approaches to particular underlying diseases, improving patients' overall quality of life. Furthermore, preventative interventions such as regular exercise, weight management, and fall prevention methods are critical for preserving knee health and reducing the chance of injury and degenerative changes over time.

Overview Of How Aging Affects The Knees

Our bodies alter as we age, and our knees are especially impacted. The knee joint is a complex system made up of bones, cartilage, ligaments, and tendons that work together to give stability and support during daily activities such as walking, jogging, and bending. However, aging may have a variety of effects on the knees, including osteoarthritis, reduced mobility, and an increased risk of injury.

One of the most noticeable symptoms of aging on the knees is the progressive wearing out of the cartilage. Cartilage is a hard, rubbery membrane that coats the ends of the bones in the knee joint, creating a smooth surface for easy movement. As we age, cartilage may degenerate due to regular wear and tear, resulting in osteoarthritis. Osteoarthritis is a degenerative joint condition that causes knee pain, stiffness, and swelling, making it difficult to walk normally.

Another factor contributing to knee difficulties as we age is the weakening of the muscles and ligaments that surround the knee joint. The muscles and ligaments support the knee and allow it to move smoothly. However, as we age, these components lose strength and flexibility, making the knee joint less stable and more susceptible to damage. Growing older, our bones tend to lose density, a disease known as osteoporosis. Osteoporosis weakens the bones of the knee joint, making them more prone to fractures and other problems.

Another typical concern associated with aging is the collection of fluid in the knee joint, which causes swelling and pain. This may be caused by several circumstances, including arthritis, injury, or excessive knee joint activity. The aging process may have a considerable influence on the knees, causing several problems that can impair mobility and quality of life. However, some things may be done to assist reduce these consequences and keep the knees healthy and functioning for as long as feasible.

Regular activity is one of the most essential methods to keep your knees healthy as you get older. Exercise helps to strengthen the muscles that surround the knee joint, increasing stability and lowering the chance of injury. It also helps to preserve the knee joint's flexibility and range of motion, which may assist relieve stiffness and discomfort.

Another important aspect of preserving knee health is keeping a healthy weight. Excess weight increases strain on the knees, which may lead to wear and tear and an increased chance of developing osteoarthritis. Maintaining a healthy weight via a balanced diet and regular exercise may help lessen the pressure on your knees and keep them in good condition.

In addition to exercise and weight control, practicing proper posture and body mechanics may help to prevent knee discomfort. Avoiding activities that cause excessive stress on the knees, such as prolonged kneeling or crouching, may also help avoid knee injuries. As we age, changes in joint fluid composition may occur, resulting in reduced lubrication inside the knee joint. This lack of lubrication may cause greater friction between the bones, aggravating soreness and stiffness.

The aging process often results in a decline in total physical activity levels, which may exacerbate knee difficulties. Reduced exercise levels may cause muscular weakening and lack of flexibility, which can worsen pre-existing knee problems and increase the risk of injury. A sedentary lifestyle may also lead to weight gain, which puts additional strain on the knee joints and increases the risk of developing osteoarthritis.

In addition to physiological changes, genetics, past injuries, and lifestyle choices may all influence how the knees age. People with a family history of osteoarthritis, for example, may be more likely to have knee difficulties as they become older. Similarly, prior knee injuries, such as ligament tears or fractures, might raise the risk of developing arthritis or other degenerative disorders in the knee joint later in life. Certain lifestyle variables, such as smoking and poor diet, might influence knee health. Smoking has been related to increased inflammation and reduced blood flow, which may lead to cartilage degradation and speed up the onset of knee osteoarthritis. Similarly, a diet strong in processed foods and sugar may cause inflammation in the body, thereby exacerbating knee pain and stiffness.

Despite these limitations, various treatments may help reduce the effects of aging on the knees while also promoting overall knee health. In addition to regular exercise and weight control, there are other therapy options available to assist manage knee discomfort and increase mobility. These treatments may involve physical therapy, medication, injections, and, in rare situations, surgery.

Physical therapy may be especially effective for seniors with knee discomfort since it focuses on strengthening the muscles around the knee joint, increasing flexibility, and teaching good body mechanics to lessen pressure on the knees. Modalities such as heat treatment, cold therapy, and ultrasound may also be utilized to reduce pain and inflammation in the knee joint.

Individuals with more serious knee issues, such as advanced osteoarthritis or considerable structural damage, may need surgical procedures such as knee replacement surgery. Knee replacement surgery removes damaged components of the knee joint and replaces them with artificial implants to restore function and relieve discomfort.

In conclusion, although aging may cause many changes in the knees that can lead to discomfort and decreased mobility, there are several treatments available to assist manage knee pain and maintain overall knee health. Seniors may help lessen the effects of aging on their knees by being active, keeping a healthy weight, and obtaining proper medical treatment as required.

Important Of Exercise For Treating Knee Discomfort

Exercise is essential for alleviating knee discomfort, particularly in seniors. As we age, our joints, particularly our knees, break down due to normal wear and tear, resulting in disorders such as osteoarthritis. While it may seem paradoxical to exercise while suffering from knee discomfort, the appropriate activities may help relieve pain and improve joint function.

1. **Strengthens Muscles:** One of the leading causes of knee discomfort is weakness of the muscles around the knee joint. Regular exercise, particularly strength training, helps to develop these muscles, offering more support and stability to the knee joint. Stronger muscles may also absorb stress and relieve strain on the knee joint during movement.

2. **Improves Flexibility and Range of Motion:** Stretching exercises may help minimize knee joint stiffness. Increased flexibility may also aid with range of motion, making it simpler to carry out everyday tasks without pain or discomfort.

3. **Maintains Knee Health:** Exercise promotes the circulation of synovial fluid, which lubricates the joint and decreases friction between the bones. This may help to lessen

inflammation and discomfort caused by illnesses such as arthritis.

4. **Weight Management:** Being overweight or obese may place additional strain on the knee joint, resulting in greater discomfort and damage. Regular exercise, paired with a nutritious diet, may aid in weight management, lowering pressure on the knees and improving overall joint health.

5. **Reduces the Risk of Falls:** Exercise may help seniors develop strong muscles and improve their balance, which can help minimize the risk of falls. Falls may result in significant injuries, including fractures, which can aggravate knee discomfort.

6. **Improves Mood and Mental Health:** Chronic pain, particularly knee pain, may have a major influence on mental health. Exercise has been found to produce endorphins, which are natural pain relievers and mood boosters. Regular exercise may help decrease stress, anxiety, and sadness, all of which are frequent among those suffering from chronic pain.

7. **Encourages Independence:** Maintaining mobility and independence is critical for elders. Seniors who exercise may improve their strength, flexibility, and balance, allowing them to continue doing everyday jobs and activities without the aid of others.

8. Improves Quality of Life: Finally, regular exercise may greatly enhance the quality of life for those who have knee discomfort. Exercise enables people to stay active and involved in life by lowering pain, increasing mobility, and boosting general well-being.

Finally, exercise is an essential component of senior knee pain management. It strengthens muscles, increases flexibility and range of motion, maintains joint health, manages weight, lowers the risk of falls, improves mood and mental health, promotes independence, and improves overall quality of life. Before beginning any new workout routine, particularly if you have pre-existing knee concerns, contact with a healthcare expert to confirm that the exercises are safe and suitable for your situation.

CHAPTER 2: BENEFITS OF EXERCISE FOR SENIORS

Discussion On The Multiple Advantages Of Regular Exercise For Seniors

Regular exercise has several advantages for elders, including improved physical, mental, and emotional well-being. Physical exercise may improve general health and quality of life, particularly as people age. Staying active has several benefits, including improved cardiovascular health, happiness, and cognitive performance.

One of the most important advantages of regular exercise for seniors is the preservation of physical health. People gradually lose muscle mass and bone density as they age, which causes frailty and an increased risk of falls and fractures. However, strength training and weight-bearing activities may assist in offsetting these effects, boosting muscle development and bone strength. Strong muscles also improve joint health, lowering the risk of acquiring illnesses like osteoarthritis.

Regular exercise is essential for preserving cardiovascular health. Aerobic exercises like walking, swimming, and cycling strengthen the heart and enhance circulation. This may reduce the risk of heart disease, stroke, and high blood pressure, all of which are increasingly common with age. Exercise also helps to manage chronic illnesses like diabetes by lowering blood sugar levels and increasing insulin sensitivity.

In addition to physical health, exercise provides important mental and emotional advantages to seniors. Staying active may improve cognitive function while lowering the chances of cognitive decline and dementia. Physical exercise causes the brain to produce chemicals that encourage the formation of new brain cells and increase connections between existing ones. This may result in improved memory, sharper reasoning, and general cognitive performance.

Exercise is also an effective mood enhancer. Physical exercise causes the release of endorphins, neurotransmitters that enhance pleasure and well-being. This may help relieve sadness and anxiety symptoms, which are frequent in older persons. Regular exercise may also help with sleep quality, which is important for general mental health and cognitive performance.

Staying active may help seniors enhance their overall quality of life by increasing their capacity to do everyday tasks. Older persons may continue to live freely and engage in activities they like if their strength, flexibility, and balance remain intact. This may help to increase a sense of purpose and satisfaction while minimizing feelings of isolation and loneliness.

Social connection is a key part of exercise for elders. Participating in group exercise classes or walking groups allows you to interact with people, which reduces feelings of loneliness and improves mental health. Social interaction has been related to a decreased risk of cognitive decline and higher emotional well-being.

To get the most out of physical activity, seniors should do a range of exercises that concentrate on strength, flexibility, balance, and cardiovascular fitness. It is recommended that you consult with a healthcare physician before beginning a new fitness plan, particularly if you have any pre-existing health concerns. Regular exercise may help seniors enhance their physical health, emotional well-being, and general quality of life.

How Exercise Can Help Relieve Knee Pain And Improve Mobility

Exercise is an effective strategy for relieving knee discomfort and increasing general mobility, particularly in seniors. While it may seem paradoxical to move more when you have knee pain, frequent and adequate exercise may strengthen the muscles surrounding the knee, improve joint flexibility, and decrease inflammation, all of which contribute to pain alleviation and increased mobility.

Exercise may help reduce knee discomfort by strengthening the muscles that support the knee joint. The quadriceps, hamstrings, and calf muscles are responsible for stabilizing the knee and absorbing trauma during movement. When these muscles are weak, the knee joint is subjected to higher stress, which causes discomfort and probable damage. Seniors may enhance muscular strength and endurance by doing exercises that target these muscle groups, such as leg lifts, squats, and lunges, which reduce pressure on the knee joint and alleviate discomfort.

Exercise improves joint flexibility and range of motion, which is especially good for seniors with knee discomfort. Stiffness in the knee joint may cause pain and restricted motion. Stretching exercises, such as hamstring and calf stretches, may help release tight muscles and increase flexibility, enabling the knee joint to move more smoothly and comfortably.

In addition to strengthening muscles and increasing flexibility, exercise may help decrease inflammation in the knee joint. Low-impact cardiovascular workouts, such as swimming and cycling, increase blood flow to the joints, which reduces inflammation and promotes healing. Furthermore, regular exercise may help you maintain a healthy weight, which is vital for minimizing the pressure on your knee joint and relieving discomfort caused by disorders like osteoarthritis.

Another significant advantage of exercise for seniors suffering from knee discomfort is increased general mobility. Mobility refers to the capacity to move freely and effortlessly, which includes tasks like walking, climbing stairs, and rising from a sitting posture. When knee discomfort restricts movement, seniors may become more sedentary, which may cause more stiffness and weakening in the muscles around the knee joint. Regular exercise may help seniors improve their general mobility, making it simpler to complete everyday tasks and preserve independence.

It's crucial to realize that not all workouts are appropriate for seniors experiencing knee discomfort. High-impact sports like jogging and leaping may aggravate knee pain and should be avoided. Instead, elders should concentrate on low-impact workouts that are easy on their joints, such as swimming, cycling, and strolling. Furthermore, before beginning any new fitness plan, contact with a healthcare practitioner, particularly if you already have knee concerns.

In conclusion, exercise is an effective technique for relieving knee discomfort and enhancing general mobility in seniors. Exercise may help seniors manage knee discomfort while also strengthening muscles, increasing flexibility, and lowering inflammation. With the help of healthcare experts, seniors may create a safe and effective fitness plan that suits their specific requirements and enhances their quality of life.

Introduction To The Concept Of Functional Fitness

Functional fitness has arisen as a pillar of modern exercise philosophy, stressing exercises that imitate real-life activities and increase an individual's capacity to do daily chores with ease and efficiency. Unlike standard gym workouts, which often isolate individual muscle groups, functional fitness programs focus on exercises that activate numerous muscle groups at the same time, developing total strength, mobility, and coordination. This comprehensive approach to fitness not only improves physical performance but also lowers the chance of injury and improves quality of life, especially for seniors and those with mobility issues.

At its foundation, functional fitness is based on the concept of functional movement patterns, which are motions that closely match everyday tasks. Squatting, lifting, pushing, pulling, bending, and twisting are all examples of motions that we do daily without even recognizing them. Functional fitness strives to increase an individual's ability to do these tasks safely and effectively, both inside and outside the gym, by including workouts that simulate these natural movement patterns.

Key Elements of Functional Fitness

Functional fitness programs often include a range of exercises and training methods to address various elements of physical function. *Some significant components are:*

1. **Strength Training:** Functional strength training focuses on complex movements that activate many muscular groups at once, such as squats, lunges, deadlifts, and overhead presses. These exercises increase muscular strength, endurance, and coordination, allowing the body to undertake everyday actions like lifting, carrying, and pushing.

2. **Mobility and Flexibility:** Mobility exercises attempt to increase joint range of motion and flexibility, resulting in smoother, more fluid movement patterns. These exercises might include dynamic stretches, foam rolling, and mobility drills that target particular joints and muscle groups. Increased mobility lowers the risk of stiffness and injury while also improving posture and movement efficiency.

3. **Balance and Stability Training:** Functional fitness programs often include exercises that require balance and stability, such as single-leg motions, Bosu ball exercises, and proprioceptive drills. Improving balance and stability not only lowers the chance of falls and injuries, but also boosts general fitness and coordination.

4. **Core Strength and Stability:** A strong and stable core is required to maintain appropriate posture, support the spine, and transmit force between the upper and lower bodies. Planks, bridges, and rotational exercises are examples of functional core workouts that target the deep stabilizing muscles of the belly, lower back, and pelvis.

5. **Cardiovascular Conditioning:** While traditional cardio exercises like running and cycling have their uses, functional fitness programs frequently include more dynamic and varied cardiovascular activities, such as interval training, circuit workouts, and functional movements like kettlebell swings and battle ropes. These workouts enhance cardiovascular endurance, engage various muscle groups, and increase functional ability.

The Benefits Of Functional Fitness

Functional fitness provides several advantages to people of all ages and fitness levels:

1. **Improved Functional Capacity:** By training movement patterns that are relevant to everyday life, functional fitness improves an individual's capacity to do daily tasks with increased ease and efficiency. This might range from carrying groceries and climbing stairs to playing with grandkids and engaging in leisure sports.

2. **Reduced Risk of Injury:** Functional fitness programs stress optimal movement mechanics, joint alignment, and muscle activation, lowering the risk of strains, sprains, and other musculoskeletal problems. Functional fitness corrects imbalances and compensates for deficits by strengthening muscles and improving mobility, hence increasing general resilience and injury avoidance.

3. **Improved Quality of Life:** Regular involvement in functional fitness activities enhances physical function, mobility, and general well-being, enabling people to live an active and independent lifestyle as they become older. Functional fitness promotes energy, confidence, and self-efficacy, resulting in a better quality of life and increased pleasure in everyday activities.

4. **Versatility and Accessibility:** Functional fitness activities may be tailored to individual requirements, preferences, and fitness levels, making them suitable for individuals of all ages and abilities. Functional fitness programs, whether done at home, in a gym, or outside, may be customized to meet individual objectives, time limits, and equipment availability.

5. **Long-Term Health and Wellness:** Regular involvement in functional fitness activities improves physical resilience, metabolic health, and functional independence. Functional fitness promotes lifespan and overall health by addressing important fitness components such as strength, mobility, balance, and cardiovascular endurance.

Functional fitness reflects a paradigm change in exercise philosophy, stressing movements that are directly applicable to everyday tasks and increase an individual's functional ability and quality of life. Functional fitness programs assist people of all ages and fitness levels by including a wide range of exercises that target strength, mobility, balance, and cardiovascular health. Whether you want to improve your sports performance, avoid injury, or just live an active and independent lifestyle, functional fitness offers a varied and accessible approach to physical health and well-being.

CHAPTER 3: SAFETY CONSIDERATIONS

Tips For Safe Exercise As A Senior With Knee Pain

Exercising properly as a senior with knee pain is critical for preserving mobility, controlling pain, and avoiding future injuries. While regular physical activity is healthy, exercise should be approached with prudence and following particular instructions to safeguard your knees.

Here are some guidelines for exercising safely as a senior with knee pain:

1. **Consult Your Doctor:** Before beginning any fitness program, speak with your doctor, particularly if you have knee discomfort or other health issues. They may provide tailored suggestions and guarantee that exercise is safe for you.

2. **Select Low-Impact Activities:** Choose low-impact activities that are easy on the knees, such as swimming, water aerobics, cycling, and walking. These exercises may

assist improve cardiovascular fitness and develop muscles without placing too much pressure on the knees.

3. **Warm Up Properly:** Always warm up before working out to prepare your muscles and joints for movement. Begin with mild motions, such as walking or marching in place, to improve blood flow and flexibility in the knee.

4. **Focus on Strength and Flexibility:** Include exercises to strengthen the muscles surrounding the knees, such as the quadriceps, hamstrings, and calves. In addition, consider exercises to increase knee flexibility and range of motion.

5. **Use Proper Form:** When exercising, pay attention to your form to prevent placing too much pressure on your knees. Use good technique and avoid overextending or locking your knees when exercising.

6. **Begin Slowly and Progress Gradually:** Begin with low-intensity workouts, gradually increasing time and intensity as your strength and endurance develop. Listen to your body and don't push yourself too much, particularly if you're in pain.

7. **Listen to Your Body:** Notice how your knees feel during and after activity. If you feel pain, swelling, or discomfort, cease your activities and rest. Continuing to exercise despite discomfort might result in greater harm.

8. **Use Proper Equipment:** When exercising, use supportive and well-fitting shoes that will cushion and stabilize your knees. If required, utilize knee braces or supports to protect your knees when exercising.

9. **Keep Hydrated:** Drink lots of water before, during, and after your workout to keep hydrated. Proper hydration is critical for joint health and may help lessen the likelihood of cramping and muscle strains.

10. **Cool Down Properly:** After exercising, spend a few minutes stretching gently. This may assist in avoiding stiffness and lower the chance of injury.

11. **Change Exercises as Needed:** If you have difficulties or pain with a particular exercise, change it to meet your requirements. For example, you may do seated versions of workouts or utilize resistance bands for light strength training.

12. **Listen to Your Healthcare Practitioner:** Adhere to any particular advice or instructions made by your healthcare practitioner or physical therapist. They can create an exercise program that is tailored to your specific requirements and assist you in exercising safely while dealing with knee discomfort.

In conclusion, exercising safely as a senior with knee discomfort requires prudence, good technique, and paying attention to your body's cues. By following these guidelines, you may get the advantages of exercise while preserving your knees and general health.

The Need For Proper Warm-Up And Cool-Down Routines

Proper warm-up and cool-down exercises are critical components of every training program, regardless of age or fitness level. These habits are critical in preparing the body for physical activity, improving performance, avoiding injuries, and encouraging recovery.

Warm-Up: Readying the Body for Action

A warm-up is a set of mild exercises conducted before more intensive physical activity. The basic goal of a warm-up is to gradually raise heart rate, blood supply to muscles, and body temperature. A warm-up prepares the body physically and psychologically for the demands of exercise.

One of the primary advantages of a good warm-up is injury avoidance. When the body is cold and unprepared, abrupt and strong physical activity may stretch muscles, ligaments, and tendons, resulting in strains, sprains, and tears. A progressive warm-up, on the other hand, helps muscles to relax and joints to move more easily, lowering the chance of injury.

A warm-up increases flexibility and range of motion, which are necessary for executing exercises with good form and technique.

Improved flexibility not only lowers the chance of injury but also improves athletic performance by enabling muscles to create more force and power when exercising.

A warm-up also helps to prepare the mind for physical activity. It allows people to concentrate their attention, imagine their next exercise, and psychologically prepare for the physical obstacles ahead. This mental preparation may help you focus, stay motivated, and perform better throughout your workout.

A typical warm-up regimen may involve modest aerobic exercises like running, cycling, or brisk walking to raise the heart rate and enhance blood flow. Dynamic stretching exercises that entail moving through a complete range of motion may also be used to better prepare the muscles and joints for activities.

Cool-Down: Aiding Recovery and Relaxation

Just as a warm-up prepares the body for exercise, a cool-down program assists the body in transitioning from effort to rest and recuperation. Cooling down after exercise is critical for improving muscular relaxation, minimizing muscle pain, and avoiding post-workout stiffness.

Muscles contract regularly during activity, causing metabolic waste such as lactic acid to build in the muscular tissues. A good cool-down assists in the clearance of toxic metabolites by increasing circulation and lymphatic drainage, hence minimizing muscular tiredness and pain.

A cool-down helps control heart rate and blood pressure, gradually returning them to their pre-exercise levels. This progressive decrease in heart rate and blood pressure helps to avoid dizziness, lightheadedness, and other possible cardiovascular concerns that may develop when the body transitions too fast from high-intensity activity to rest.

A cool-down not only delivers bodily advantages but also allows for mental rest and introspection. It enables people to step away from the intensity of their exercise, relax, and mentally celebrate their accomplishments. This moment of relaxation may assist to decrease stress, improve mood, and boost general well-being.

A typical cool-down practice may include low-intensity cardiovascular exercises like walking or mild cycling to gradually drop heart rate and improve circulation. Static stretching exercises, which hold muscles in a prolonged posture without movement, may also be used to relieve stress and improve flexibility.

To summarize, adequate warm-up and cool-down routines are critical components of a safe and successful exercise regimen. A comprehensive warm-up prepares the body for physical action by boosting blood flow, improving flexibility, and psychologically preparing for the workout. A well-executed cool-down, on the other hand, helps with recovery by inducing muscular relaxation, lowering pain, and assisting in the clearance of metabolic waste. By including these exercises in your workout program, you may improve performance, avoid injuries, and enhance general health and well-being.

Guidelines For Listening To Your Body And Avoiding Overexertion

Listening to your body and avoiding overexertion are critical components of any workout plan, particularly for seniors with knee discomfort. Overexertion may cause injuries and setbacks in your fitness goal. Understanding your body's signals and understanding when to push and when to relax is essential for safely and efficiently managing knee discomfort.

1. **Understanding Your Body's Signals:** Your body communicates with you via a variety of signs, including pain, discomfort, exhaustion, and difficulty breathing. It is critical to pay attention to these indications, particularly while exercising with knee discomfort. Differentiate between typical muscular weariness and discomfort that suggests an injury. Pay attention to your body's signals and change your exercise level appropriately.

2. **Begin Slowly and Progressively:** When starting an exercise program, start with low-intensity exercises and progressively increase the intensity and length as your fitness improves. This slow approach helps your body to adjust to the increased demands, lowering the likelihood of overexertion and damage. Avoid the temptation to take on too much too quickly, which may lead to fatigue and setbacks.

3. **Use the Speak Test:** The speak test is a simple approach to determine how intense your workout is. Moderate-intensity exercise should allow you to talk in short phrases but not sing. If you're too out of breath to speak, you may have overexerted yourself. Adjust your intensity to maintain a comfortable level of effort.

4. **Monitor Your Heart Rate:** Tracking your heart rate may help you maintain a safe and effective workout intensity. Use a heart rate monitor or check your pulse often when exercising. Aim for a heart rate that is appropriate for your age and fitness level. Exceeding this zone may indicate overexertion.

5. **Pay Attention to Joint and Muscle Pain:** While some discomfort during exercise is expected, acute or prolonged pain in your joints or muscles should not be overlooked. If you feel discomfort, discontinue your activities and rest. Continuing to exercise despite discomfort might result in greater harm. If you are experiencing chronic discomfort, consult with a healthcare expert.

6. **Rest and Recovery:** Rest is an important part of any training routine. Allow your body to rest between sessions to avoid overtraining and encourage muscle recovery. Adequate rest may also help you avoid burnout and stay inspired to continue exercising.

7. **Stay Hydrated and Fuel Your Body:** Proper hydration and nutrition are essential for sustaining your body throughout activity. Drink lots of water before, during, and after your exercise to keep hydrated. Fuel your body with healthy meals that supply the energy and nutrition it needs for activity and recuperation.

8. **Listen to Your Mind:** Overexertion may also be avoided by paying attention to your mental condition. Pay attention to how you feel psychologically when exercising. If you're feeling excessively tired, apprehensive, or agitated, it might be a hint that you should relax. Exercise should be fun and stimulating, not depleting.

To summarize, listening to your body and avoiding overexertion is critical for properly managing knee discomfort during exercise. You may get the advantages of exercise while lowering your risk of injury by paying attention to your body's cues, beginning gently and progressively. Remember to relax, remain hydrated, and nourish your body appropriately to help you achieve your fitness objectives. If you're not sure how to exercise safely with knee discomfort, speak with a healthcare practitioner or a qualified fitness trainer for specialized advice.

CHAPTER 4: RANGE OF MOTION EXERCISES

Gentle Exercises To Enhance Flexibility And Range Of Motion In The Knees

Maintaining knee flexibility and range of motion is critical for general mobility and joint health, particularly for seniors who suffer from knee pain or stiffness. Gentle exercises that target the knee joints may help relieve pain, enhance function, and avoid additional mobility restrictions.

1. Knee Circles

1. Stand upright, feet together, knees bent.
2. Place your hands on your knees and gently spin them in tiny circles.
3. Finish one set and then move to the other way.

2. Quadriceps Stretch

1. If you can stand steadily, grasp onto a chair or counter or put your hand on a wall. You may practice this workout while lying on your stomach or side.
2. Bend the knee in the leg you wish to stretch, then reach back with the same hand to grip the front of your foot. For example, if you want to extend your right leg, use your right hand.
3. With your knees close to each other, move your foot toward your buttock until you feel a slight stretch over the front of your hip and down the front of your thighs. Your knee should be aimed squarely toward the ground, not off to the side.
4. Hold the stretch for at least 15-30 seconds.
5. Repeat 2–4 times for each leg.

3. Seated Knee Flexion

1. Sit on the edge of a chair.
2. Gently slip one foot backward, bending your knee as much as possible... without pushing it. It's acceptable if your heel begins to rise off the ground.
3. Sit straight on your bottom, relax the muscles on the top of your thigh, and hold for 30 seconds.
4. Repeat the stretch 2 to 4 times on one side, gradually progressing to holding it for a minute.

5. Then swap legs and repeat the exercise 2 to 4 times on the other side.
6. Some soreness or discomfort is to be anticipated... but cease completing the workout if you experience greater pain.

4. Standing Calf Stretch

1. Stand facing a wall, hands on the wall at eye level.
2. Position the leg you wish to extend roughly a step behind the other leg.
3. Keep your back heel on the floor and bend your front knee until you feel a stretch in your back leg.
4. Hold the stretch for 15–30 seconds.

5. Leg Swings

1. Begin with standing on one leg, then swinging the other leg forth and back.
2. Start with modest swings and proceed to greater swings as tolerated.
3. Next, turn to side-to-side leg swings.

6. Heel Slide

1. Lie on the floor or in bed, with your leg flat.
2. Begin slowly sliding your heel toward your buttocks while maintaining it on the floor or bed. Your knee will start to bend.
3. Continue to slip your heel and bend your knee until you feel some discomfort and pressure within your knee.
4. Hold this posture for about 6 seconds.
5. Return your heel to the floor or bed, ensuring that your leg is straight.

Incorporating simple knee flexibility and range of motion exercises into your daily routine may have a major impact on joint health and mobility, particularly for seniors suffering knee discomfort or stiffness. By completing these exercises daily, you may assist relieve pain, avoid additional mobility limits, and maintain an active lifestyle. Remember to listen to your body, start cautiously, and check with a healthcare expert if you have any concerns or pre-existing knee difficulties. With persistence and perseverance, you may enhance your knees' flexibility and function, thus improving your overall quality of life.

The Significance Of Retaining Joint Mobility For Pain Alleviation

Maintaining joint mobility is critical for pain treatment, particularly for seniors with knee discomfort. Joint mobility refers to a joint's capacity to move freely over its whole range of motion. When joints are stiff or limited in their mobility, it may cause discomfort, suffering, and reduced functioning. This is especially true for the knee joint, which is very prone to wear and strain over time.

One of the most essential reasons to maintain joint mobility for pain treatment is that it helps to avoid the development of disorders like osteoarthritis. Osteoarthritis is a degenerative joint condition that mostly affects the knees, resulting in pain, stiffness, and edema. By keeping the joints mobile and flexible, the chance of developing osteoarthritis and other joint-related disorders decreases.

Maintaining joint mobility may assist in reducing pain and discomfort. Allowing joints to move freely may assist in lubricating the joint surfaces and minimize friction, which can help to alleviate discomfort. Furthermore, maintaining mobility might assist in enhancing the strength and flexibility of the muscles that surround the joint, resulting in greater support and stability.

Joint mobility also plays a vital part in maintaining total joint health. When joints are immobile or have limited mobility, toxins and waste materials accumulate in the joint area, contributing to inflammation and discomfort. Maintaining joint mobility promotes improved circulation and the elimination of toxic chemicals, which may help to minimize pain and enhance joint health.

In addition to the physical advantages, preserving joint mobility may improve mental health. Chronic pain may hurt one's mental health, causing irritation, worry, and sadness. Improving joint mobility and lowering discomfort may assist in enhancing mood and general quality of life.

There are numerous approaches to maintaining joint mobility for pain management. One of the most effective approaches is to engage in regular exercise. Exercise improves flexibility, strength, and range of motion, which may help keep joints flexible and relieve discomfort. Low-impact workouts like swimming, cycling, and yoga are especially good for preserving joint mobility without placing too much load on them.

Stretching is a vital part of preserving joint mobility. Stretching promotes flexibility and range of motion, which may assist in alleviating stiffness and discomfort. Stretching should be done often and carefully, since overstretching may cause damage.

Maintaining a healthy weight is also beneficial to joint health and mobility. Excess weight puts additional pressure on the joints, especially the knees, which may cause pain and discomfort. Maintaining a healthy weight with a balanced diet and regular exercise may lower the risk of joint disorders and enhance mobility.

To summarize, preserving joint mobility is critical for pain management, especially for seniors with knee discomfort. Maintaining joint mobility and flexibility may assist to avoid joint disorders, relieve current pain, and enhance overall joint health. Regular exercise, stretching, and keeping a healthy weight are all essential for preserving joint mobility and minimizing discomfort.

CHAPTER 5: STRENGTHENING EXERCISES

Introduction To Strength Training Routines That Are Especially Good For Seniors With Knee Pain

Strength training activities designed specifically for seniors with knee pain may be a vital component of a complete strategy for controlling pain, increasing mobility, and improving overall quality of life.

Sarcopenia refers to the normal reduction in muscular mass and strength that occurs as we age. This muscle loss might increase knee discomfort because weakening muscles may fail to appropriately support and stabilize the knee joint. Strength training, also known as resistance training, is completing exercises that put the muscles against resistance, encouraging muscular development and increasing strength.

For seniors with knee discomfort, strength training provides numerous significant benefits:

1. **Improved Joint Stability:** Strengthening the muscles that surround the knee joint may assist increase stability and minimize the chance of injury or pain.

2. **Enhanced Functionality:** Stronger muscles allow for improved movement control and coordination, which facilitates everyday tasks and promotes independence.

3. **Pain Reduction:** Strengthening the muscles surrounding the knee may help distribute forces more evenly throughout the joint, thereby relieving pain and lowering pressure on sensitive tissues.

4. **Better Joint Protection:** Stronger muscles function as protective buffers for the knee joint, absorbing stress and mitigating the effects of repeated motions.

Important Considerations for Strength Training

Before starting a strength training program, seniors with knee discomfort should examine the following things to guarantee safety and effectiveness:

1. **Consultation with Healthcare Professional:** Before beginning any new fitness plan, you should check with a healthcare professional, especially if you have pre-existing knee difficulties or medical concerns.

2. **Good Form and Technique:** Learning good workout techniques is critical for increasing benefits while lowering the chance of injury. Consider working with a skilled fitness expert to verify you are doing workouts properly.

3. **Begin Slowly and Progress Progressively:** Begin with minimal resistance and progressively increase intensity as your strength and comfort improve. Avoid pushing through discomfort and instead heed your body's messages.

4. **Individualized Approach:** Tailor your strength training program to your unique requirements, preferences, and limits. Exercises may be modified as required to suit any pain or mobility limits.

Specific Strength Training Exercises for Seniors With Knee Pain:

Here are many excellent strength training routines aimed at important muscle groups that support and stabilize the knee joint:

1. **Leg Press:** Using a leg press machine or resistance bands, sit comfortably and stretch your legs to push the weight away from you. This workout focuses on the quadriceps, hamstrings, and glutes.

2. **Leg Extensions:** Sit on a leg extension machine, knees bent at a 90-degree angle. Extend your legs and raise the weight by straightening your knees. This workout mainly works the quadriceps.

3. **Hamstring Curls:** Lie face down with your knees bent, curling the weight toward your buttocks using a leg curl machine or resistance bands. This exercise strengthens the hamstrings, which are essential for knee stabilization.

4. **Calf Raises:** Stand with your feet hip-width apart and raise to the balls of your feet, elevating your heels as high as possible. Gradually drop your heels back down. This workout specifically targets the calf muscles.

5. **Step-Ups:** Using a strong step or platform, raise one foot and pull the opposing knee up to your chest. Step back down and repeat on the other side. This exercise works the quadriceps, hamstrings, and glutes while improving balance.

6. **Wall Sits:** Stand with your back against a wall and lower your body to a seated posture, as if in an imaginary chair. Hold this posture for as long as you feel comfortable, progressively increasing the length over time. This workout develops the quadriceps and glutes.

7. **Resistance Band Workouts:** Add resistance bands to your program to execute workouts like lateral leg lifts, clamshells, and seated leg presses. These exercises give resistance in many directions and target different muscle groups around the knee.

Strength training activities designed for seniors with knee discomfort have several advantages, including greater joint stability, increased functioning, pain relief, and better joint protection. Seniors who use targeted exercises that strengthen the muscles around the knee joint may successfully manage pain, enhance mobility, and continue an active lifestyle. Strength training may be an effective strategy for increasing knee health and general well-being in older individuals when done correctly, with tailored programming and a commitment to regularity.

Tips To Gradually Increase Resistance And Intensity

Exercise resistance and intensity should be gradually increased for seniors who want to successfully treat knee discomfort while also improving general strength and mobility. Seniors may increase strength and resilience while reducing their chance of injury by gently testing their muscles and joints.

1. **Begin Slowly:** Seniors should start with exercises that are pleasant and doable, emphasizing appropriate form and technique. This might involve doing bodyweight workouts or utilizing mild resistance bands or weights.

2. **Gradually Increase Weight:** As seniors' strength increases, they may gradually increase the amount of weight or resistance utilized in their workouts. This may be accomplished by increasing the weight increments or utilizing resistance bands with greater tension levels.

3. **Monitor Your Comfort and Fatigue Levels:** Seniors should pay attention to how their bodies feel during and after exercise. Gradually increasing resistance should be demanding but not too painful or exhausting. If the workouts become too challenging, you may need to temporarily lower the weight or intensity.

4. **Focus on Appropriate Form:** Maintaining appropriate form is critical for avoiding injury and increasing the efficacy of exercise. Seniors should emphasize quality over quantity, ensuring that each exercise is performed correctly over the whole range of motion.

5. **Progressive Overload:** The progressive overload theory entails progressively increasing the demands imposed on the body over time to generate ongoing increases in strength and fitness. This may be accomplished by gradually increasing the weight, repetitions, or length of the workouts.

6. **Use Range:** Including a range of exercises that target various muscle groups will help you avoid plateaus and keep sessions interesting. Seniors should include workouts that target the quadriceps, hamstrings, calves, and other muscles around the knees to create balanced strength and stability.

7. **Listen to Your Body:** Seniors should pay attention to their bodies signals and alter their fitness routines appropriately. It is critical to discern between typical muscular weariness and discomfort that might suggest an injury. If you are suffering from chronic or increasing discomfort, you should visit a healthcare expert.

8. **Rest and Recovery:** Muscles need enough rest and recovery to mend and develop stronger. Seniors should include rest days in their fitness regimen and emphasize activities that

promote relaxation and stress reduction, such as moderate stretching or meditation.

9. **Consider Functional Motions:** Functional exercises replicate daily motions and might be especially effective for seniors who want to enhance knee function and minimize discomfort. Squats, lunges, and step-ups are examples of exercises that strengthen the muscles needed in tasks such as walking and ascending stairs.

10. **Consult with an Expert:** Before beginning or changing an exercise plan, seniors should speak with a healthcare expert, such as a physical therapist or personal trainer who has worked with older persons. These specialists may give tailored advice and suggestions depending on the individual's requirements and ability.

In conclusion, gradually increasing resistance and intensity in exercise is an important component of controlling knee discomfort and improving overall strength and mobility in seniors. Starting carefully, concentrating on appropriate technique, and progressively pushing the body over time may help seniors increase strength, decrease discomfort, and improve their quality of life. Listen to your body, emphasize safety, and seek expert advice as required to create a safe and successful fitness regimen.

CHAPTER 6: BALANCE AND STABILITY TRAINING

The Significance Of Balance And Stability Exercises In Reducing Falls And Enhancing Knee Function

Exercises that improve balance and stability are particularly important for seniors' general health and well-being. These exercises not only assist in reducing falls but also enhance knee function, which is critical for retaining independence and quality of life as we age.

Balance and stability exercises are vital for seniors because they help avoid falls. Falls are a major worry for older persons, with one in every four people aged 65 and above falling each year. Falls may cause catastrophic injuries such as hip fractures and brain damage, limiting a person's capacity to live freely. Seniors who improve their balance and stability may lower their chance of falling while still maintaining their mobility and independence.

Balance and stability exercises also assist in enhancing knee function, which is necessary for leading an active lifestyle. As we age, our joints may stiffen and become less flexible, causing pain and limiting movement, especially in the knees. Seniors may minimize pain and stiffness by strengthening the muscles around the knee joint, as well as increasing balance and stability, enabling them to move more freely and participate in enjoyable activities.

Balance and stability exercises may help you gain overall strength and flexibility, which are essential for proper posture and avoiding musculoskeletal ailments. These exercises work essential muscle groups including the quadriceps, hamstrings, and calf muscles, which support the knee joint and absorb stress during movement. Seniors who exercise these muscles may lessen pressure on their knee joints and enhance their overall function.

Balance and stability exercises also improve proprioception, or the body's capacity to perceive its location in space. Proprioception is essential for maintaining balance and coordination, particularly as we age. Balance exercises may help seniors improve their proprioception, making it simpler for them to manage uneven terrain and prevent falls.

Balance and stability exercises assist seniors not only physically, but also mentally and emotionally. These activities may help boost mood and alleviate typical anxiety and depression symptoms in older persons. Seniors who keep active and participate in regular exercise may retain a happy attitude and enhance their overall quality of life.

general, balance and stability exercises are critical for minimizing falls in seniors, increasing knee function, and preserving general health and well-being. Seniors who include these activities in their daily routine may minimize their chance of falling, enhance their mobility and independence, and have a better quality of life as they age.

Demonstrations Of Exercises To Enhance Balance, Proprioception, And Coordination

Improving balance, proprioception, and coordination is critical for seniors, particularly those with knee discomfort. These abilities not only improve mobility and lower the danger of falling, but they also contribute to total functional independence and quality of life. In this tutorial, we'll look at several exercises created particularly for these regions, with step-by-step examples and explanations to help seniors implement them into their regular routines.

Exercise Demonstrations

1. Single Leg Stance

1. For added support, stand near a strong chair or countertop.
2. Lift one foot off the ground and balance on the other leg.
3. Hold the posture for 10–30 seconds before switching legs.
4. Maintain a tall posture while utilizing your core muscles for stability.

2. Tandem Walk

1. Locate a clean route where you can walk in a straight manner.
2. Place one foot exactly in front of the other, with the heel of the front foot touching the toes of the rear foot.
3. Walk forward in this way for 10-20 steps while keeping balance and coordination.
4. If necessary, utilize a wall or railing as support.

3. Heel-to-Toe Walk

1. Start by standing with your feet together.
2. Take a step forward, bringing the heel of one foot exactly in front of the toes of the other.
3. Continue walking in a straight line, keeping the heel-to-toe rhythm.
4. Maintain a steady pace and use your core muscles for balance.

4. Standing Leg Swings

1. To maintain balance, stand near a wall or firm support.
2. Swing one leg forth and backward in a controlled manner while keeping a straight stance.
3. Swing 10-15 times with each leg, progressively increasing the range of motion as you feel more comfortable.
4. To test your balance and stability, swing your leg from side to side.

5. Tai Chi-Inspired Movements

1. Stand shoulder-width apart, with knees slightly bent.
2. Transfer your weight to one leg while elevating the other foot off the ground.
3. Slowly stretch the elevated leg to the side and then back to the center.
4. Repeat on the other side, moving with fluidity and control.
5. As you gain proficiency, integrate arm motions to improve coordination.

6. Balance Board Exercises

1. Position your feet hip-width apart on a balancing board or padded surface.
2. Use your core muscles to stay stable while the board moves under you.
3. Practice moving your weight side to side and front to back, gradually increasing the difficulty.
4. Begin with short periods, gradually increasing to longer sessions as your balance improves.

By adding these exercises for improving balance, proprioception, and coordination into your daily routine, you may increase your general mobility, minimize your chance of falling, and keep your independence as you age. Remember to start cautiously, remain consistent, and emphasize safety at all times. With devotion and practice, you may reap the advantages of enhanced balance and coordination far into your retirement years.

Integrating Balancing Issues Into Regular Activities

Incorporating balancing challenges into everyday activities is an important part of maintaining and increasing balance, stability, and general physical well-being, particularly for seniors and those with mobility limitations. Balance is an essential component of functional fitness and plays an important role in avoiding falls and injuries. Individuals who include balancing difficulties into their everyday routines may improve their balance abilities, strengthen supporting muscles, and increase proprioception, which is the body's capacity to detect its location in space.

One of the easiest ways to add balance issues into everyday activities is to complete regular chores while standing on one leg. For example, when brushing teeth or cleaning dishes, one may raise one foot off the ground and keep it there for as long as it is comfortable before switching to the other leg. This basic exercise increases stability and improves the muscles in the ankles, knees, and hips.

Another excellent technique to introduce balance issues is to use unstable surfaces. This may be as easy as standing on a cushion or pillow while doing something like doing clothes or watching television. The uneven surface requires the body to use fewer stabilizing muscles, which improves balance and coordination with time.

Walking heel-to-toe is a traditional balancing exercise that may be readily included in everyday walks or even when walking about the home. With each stride, place the heel of one foot squarely in front of the toes of the other, as if walking on a tightrope. This tests balance and improves coordination.

Incorporating yoga or tai chi into your regular practice may also help you achieve better balance and stability. These practices include a sequence of fluid movements and positions that need focus, coordination, and balance. Even a few minutes of yoga or tai chi every day may significantly enhance balance and well-being.

Using balance aids like a balance board or a stability ball may also help. These instruments create an unstable surface for standing on, requiring the body to activate core muscles and enhance balance. They may be used to offer a balancing challenge to everyday activities such as working at a standing desk or watching TV.

Incorporating balancing problems throughout normal activities may also improve cognitive function. Balancing requires attention and concentration, which may enhance cognitive performance and mental sharpness. This is especially crucial as we age, since cognitive decline may be a problem.

To summarize, introducing balance challenges into everyday activities is a simple yet effective strategy to enhance balance, stability, and general physical and mental health. Individuals who include short balancing exercises in their everyday routines may improve their balance abilities, lower their chance of falling, and improve their quality of life.

CHAPTER 7: LOW-IMPACT CARDIOVASCULAR EXERCISES

Overview Of The Advantages Of Cardiovascular Exercise For Knee Health

Cardiovascular exercise, sometimes known as cardio, is any activity that boosts your heart rate and improves blood circulation throughout the body. While it is usually related to improved heart health and overall fitness, it also has various knee-specific advantages. These advantages are especially relevant for the elderly and those with knee problems since they may help control pain, increase mobility, and improve overall quality of life.

1. **Strengthens Muscles Near the Knee:** Walking, cycling, and swimming are all cardiovascular workouts that help strengthen the muscles around the knee joint. Stronger muscles help to support and stabilize the knee, lowering the chance of injury and easing joint tension.

2. **Improves Joint Flexibility:** Regular cardio may increase joint flexibility, which is essential for knee health. Improved

flexibility alleviates stiffness in the knee joint and surrounding muscles, making movement simpler and more pleasant.

3. **Promotes Weight Loss:** Excess weight increases strain on the knees, resulting in greater wear and tear over time. Cardio workouts burn calories and assist in weight reduction, reducing knee strain and discomfort.

4. **Boosts Joint Lubrication:** Cardiovascular activity improves blood flow to the joints, especially the knees, which aids in the formation of synovial fluids. This fluid serves as a lubricant for the joints, decreasing friction and improving mobility.

5. **Boosts Circulation:** Proper circulation is necessary for providing oxygen and nutrients to the tissues around the knee joint. Cardiovascular activity boosts circulation, ensuring that the knee joint obtains the nutrients it needs for healing and maintenance.

6. **Reduces Inflammation:** Chronic inflammation is a prevalent concern among people who have knee problems. Cardio workouts may help decrease inflammation by increasing the production of anti-inflammatory molecules in the body, which relieves pain and swelling.

7. **Improves Cardiovascular Health:** Good cardiovascular health is important for general well-being and may have an indirect impact on knee health. A healthy heart may pump blood more effectively, resulting in better circulation and delivery of oxygen and nutrients to the knee.

8. **Boosts Mood and Mental Health:** Regular cardio has been found to improve mood while also reducing symptoms of anxiety and sadness. This is particularly important for those who have knee pain since it helps them remain motivated and optimistic about their rehabilitation.

9. **Increases Energy Levels:** Regular cardio may boost energy levels, making everyday tasks and workout regimens simpler to handle. This is especially beneficial for seniors with knee concerns, since it may enhance their general quality of life and independence.

10. **Improves Sleep:** Cardiovascular activity may help you get a better night's sleep, which is important for your overall health. Better sleep may also assist in lowering pain perception, making it simpler to treat knee discomfort.

Finally, cardiovascular activity has several advantages for knee health. Regular exercise may help manage knee discomfort by strengthening muscles, increasing flexibility, boosting weight reduction, and lowering inflammation. Incorporating a range of aerobic activities into your regimen, along with correct warm-up and cool-down routines, will help you gain these advantages while also keeping your knees healthy and strong.

Introduction To Low-Impact Exercises For Seniors With Knee Pain

Physical exercise is critical to preserving overall health and well-being, particularly as we age. However, for seniors with knee discomfort, high-impact workouts such as jogging or leaping may be difficult and can aggravate pre-existing knee problems. Low-impact workouts are a mild but effective option that provides several advantages while placing little strain on the knees. Swimming and cycling are two popular low-impact workouts for seniors dealing with knee discomfort.

Swimming is often cited as one of the finest kinds of exercise for those with knee discomfort. The buoyancy of water minimizes the effects of gravity, making motions simpler and less strenuous on the joints. This feature of water also offers light resistance, allowing muscles to be strengthened without the need for heavy weights or apparatus. Swimming works many muscle groups, including those around the knees, which helps to enhance overall strength and flexibility. Swimming is also a cardiovascular activity, which benefits the heart and lungs while burning calories and helps with weight control.

Cycling, whether on a stationary bike or outside, is another wonderful low-impact activity for seniors with knee discomfort. Cycling provides for a smooth, circular action that puts less pressure on the knees. Stationary bikes' adjustable resistance allows users to customize the intensity of their activity, making them appropriate for all fitness levels. Outdoor cycling also gives the extra advantage of fresh air and picturesque sights, making it a relaxing and pleasurable pastime. Cycling, like swimming, provides excellent cardiovascular exercise while also enhancing heart health and stamina.

Swimming and cycling provide various benefits for seniors who suffer from knee discomfort. One of the primary advantages is increased joint mobility and flexibility. These exercises use repeated actions to lubricate the joints, decreasing stiffness and improving range of motion. This is especially advantageous for seniors suffering from illnesses such as arthritis, which may restrict movement and create knee pain.

Swimming and cycling also help to strengthen the muscles surrounding the knees. Muscle strength is essential for supporting and stabilizing the knees, reducing discomfort and the risk of damage. Stronger muscles increase general balance and coordination, lowering the risk of falls, which are particularly deadly for seniors.

Swimming and cycling are low-impact activities that are easy on the joints. This makes them ideal for seniors suffering from knee pain or other joint difficulties since they reduce the chance of additional injury or discomfort. Unlike high-impact workouts, which may cause joint pain, low-impact activities are a safe and effective method to keep active and healthy.

Swimming and cycling have been shown to improve mental health in addition to their physical advantages. Exercise produces endorphins, or "feel-good" chemicals that may help alleviate stress, anxiety, and sadness. Regular physical exercise may improve mood, self-esteem, and quality of life.

Finally, swimming and cycling are wonderful low-impact sports for seniors with knee discomfort. These exercises have several advantages, including greater joint mobility, muscular strength, cardiovascular fitness, and mental well-being. Swimming or cycling may help seniors maintain an active lifestyle, manage knee discomfort, and improve their overall health and vitality.

Tips To Maintain Cardiovascular Fitness Without Exacerbating Knee Issues

Maintaining cardiovascular fitness is critical for general health, but for those with knee pain or other knee issues, finding strategies to exercise without exacerbating symptoms may be difficult. *However, some various ideas and tactics may help you maintain cardiovascular fitness and safeguard your knees:*

1. **Select Low-Impact Activities:** Choose knee-friendly activities such as swimming, water aerobics, cycling (stationary or outdoor), and elliptical exercise. These sports provide a cardiovascular workout without placing too much pressure on the knees.

2. **Focus on Form:** Proper form is vital for avoiding knee discomfort during activity. For example, while cycling, keep your knees aligned with your feet and avoid locking them out at the bottom of the pedal stroke. To decrease knee discomfort, swim using suitable methods.

3. **Gradually Increase Intensity:** Begin cautiously and gradually raise the intensity of your exercises to minimize unexpected stress on your knees. This slow escalation enables your muscles and joints to get used to the increasing effort.

4. **Use Proper Footwear:** Wearing supportive and cushioned shoes may assist lessen the impact on the knees when exercising. Look for shoes with strong arch support and cushioning in the heel and forefoot.

5. **Warm up and Cool Down:** Always start your workout with a suitable warm-up to prepare your muscles and joints for movement. After your exercise, cool down with easy stretches to retain flexibility and decrease muscular pain.

6. **Cross Train:** Include a diversity of exercises in your workout program to lessen the chance of overuse injuries. This may also help you keep active while resting your knees from high-impact activities.

7. **Listen to Your Body:** Notice how your knees feel during and after activity. If you feel pain or discomfort, stop and rest. Pushing through discomfort might result in greater harm.

8. **Use Proper Equipment:** When utilizing workout equipment like stationary cycles or elliptical machines, be sure the settings are appropriate for your physique and comfort level. This might assist in relieving tension on your knees.

9. **Maintain a Healthy Weight:** Excess weight might cause additional strain on your knees. Maintaining a healthy

weight via food and exercise may lessen the pressure on your knees while also improving your overall health.

10. **Consult a Professional:** If you experience knee discomfort or a knee issue, speak with a physical therapist or a healthcare specialist. They may provide tailored suggestions and offer direction to help you maintain cardiovascular fitness while preserving your knees.

To summarize, maintaining cardiovascular fitness without exacerbating knee issues needs a combination of selecting the ideal exercises, practicing good form, gradually increasing intensity, and listening to your body. By following these guidelines, you may remain active and improve your cardiovascular health while also preserving your knees from additional harm.

CHAPTER 8: MIND-BODY EXERCISES

Investigation Of Mind-Body Methods For Controlling Knee Pain

Mind-body therapies are well recognized for their holistic approach to health and wellness. Yoga, tai chi, meditation, and deep breathing exercises are examples of activities that stress the mind-body link. While typically used to reduce stress and improve mental health, they have also been shown to be useful in the treatment of physical problems such as knee pain.

The mind-body link is the complicated interplay between our ideas, emotions, and bodily experiences. A new study reveals that our mental and emotional states might impact how we perceive pain and how our bodies respond to it. Stress, worry, and depression, for example, may worsen pain by causing physiological reactions like muscular tension and inflammation.

Mind-body practices seek to leverage this link by encouraging relaxation, mindfulness, and emotional well-being. These practices promote inner peace and balance via gentle movements, breath exercises, and meditation, which may improve pain perception and tolerance.

Practicing Yoga To Reduce Knee Pain

Yoga, an ancient practice from India, has grown in popularity across the globe due to its multiple health advantages. When properly adjusted, yoga may be an effective technique for addressing knee discomfort. Gentle yoga postures and sequences enhance flexibility, strength, and joint stability while also relieving tension and encouraging relaxation.

Certain yoga postures, including Child's Pose, Downward-Facing Dog, and Warrior II, gently stretch the muscles surrounding the knees, improving mobility and relieving stiffness. Yoga also promotes optimal alignment and body awareness, lowering the chance of injury and improving posture, which may ease pressure on the knees.

Demonstrating Yoga for Knee Pain Relief

1. Child's Pose (Balasana)

1. Sit on your heels with your knees spaced a distance apart, and bring your head to the floor.
2. Your arms may be extended out to the front, at your side, or below your forehead.
3. Breathe in your lower back.

4. Stay in this resting stance for ranging from 30 seconds to several minutes.
5. To exit, exhale and roll up each vertebra, or return to a sitting position with a straight spine.

2. Downward Facing Dog (Adho Mukha Svanasana)

1. Get on your hands and knees. Bring your hands slightly in front of your shoulders, spread your fingers, push down with your knuckles, and tuck your toes.
2. Exhale as you raise your knees and extend your hips up and back.
3. Keep your knees slightly bent and push the backs of your thighs on the wall behind you, extending your heels toward the mat.
4. Push the base of your index fingers into the mat. Rest your neck and keep your head between your upper arms.
5. Take a breath here. As you exhale, bend your knees and drop yourself into Child's pose.

3. Warrior II (Virabhadrasana II)

1. Begin in Tadasana / Mountain pose at the front of your mat, then step back with your left leg, toes pointed slightly in.
2. Press the four corners of your feet down and tighten your legs.
3. Inhale and lift your arms parallel to the floor while keeping your shoulders down and your neck long.

4. As you exhale, bend your right knee, keeping it above your ankle. If necessary, gently modify the location of your feet and legs to achieve stability in the posture.
5. Roll the top of your thigh down to the floor on the right. To balance the movement, press down through your big toe.
6. Press the top of your left leg back and place the outside of your left foot on the floor.
7. Draw your lower abdomen forward and up, lengthening your spine. Extend through your collarbones and fingers. To correct your neck and spine, bring your chin gently in and back. Look at your right hand.
8. Hold this stance for five breaths. To exit the posture, push into your feet and straighten your legs while inhaling. Switch the alignment of your feet and repeat on the other side.

Always listen to your body and adjust your positions as required to minimize pain or strain. If you have any current knee problems, you should contact a healthcare practitioner before beginning a new workout plan.

Tai Chi For Knee Pain Relief

Tai chi, sometimes known as "moving meditation," is a mind-body exercise originated in China that blends slow, flowing motions with deep breathing and mental attention. Unlike high-impact workouts, tai chi is easy on the knees, making it a good alternative for seniors who have knee problems.

Research has shown that regular tai chi practice helps enhance balance, coordination, and strength, all of which are important for knee stability and injury prevention. Tai chi promotes relaxation and reduces stress, which helps relieve tension in the muscles and joints, resulting in less discomfort and better general well-being.

Meditation and Deep Breathing Exercises

Meditation and deep breathing techniques are effective ways to manage pain and promote calm. Mindfulness meditation, in particular, is concentrating attention on the current moment without judgment, enabling people to examine their thoughts and feelings without becoming overwhelmed by them.

Meditation may help people build a new connection with their suffering by increasing awareness and acceptance and lowering fear and resistance. Deep breathing techniques, such as diaphragmatic breathing or belly breathing, trigger the body's relaxation response, which calms the nervous system and relieves muscular tension, even in the knees.

One of the advantages of mind-body therapies is their flexibility to different lives and tastes. These activities, whether used in a formal classroom context or integrated into regular routines at home, provide flexibility and accessibility.

Seniors with knee discomfort might benefit from incorporating mind-body activities into their everyday lives in easy ways. This might involve taking brief pauses during the day for deep breathing exercises, practicing mindfulness while walking or doing housework, or attending frequent yoga or tai chi courses customized to their specific requirements.

To summarize, mind-body techniques provide a comprehensive approach to controlling knee pain by addressing the interdependence of the mind and body. Gentle exercises, breath work, meditation, and mindfulness increase relaxation, decrease stress, and improve general well-being, thus relieving knee pain and improving seniors' quality of life. Seniors who include mind-body techniques into their daily routines may empower themselves to take an active part in their pain management journey and create a stronger feeling of resilience and energy.

Mind-Body Activities May Improve General Well-Being

In today's fast-paced society, the value of holistic well-being is widely acknowledged as critical to living a healthy and satisfying life. Mind-body activities like yoga, tai chi, and mindfulness meditation have grown in popularity due to their positive effects on physical, mental, and emotional health. These activities represent the union of mind and body, providing several advantages that contribute to total well-being.

Mind-body exercises focus on the relationship between mental processes, physical motions, and breath awareness. Individuals get a better knowledge of their internal condition via purposeful practice and concentrated attention, encouraging harmony and balance within themselves and in the environment around them. Let's look at the several advantages of adding mind-body workouts into your program.

1. **Tension Reduction:** Mind-body exercises are well known for their potential to reduce tension and promote relaxation. By using slow, methodical motions and deep breathing methods, practitioners promote the body's relaxation response, which counteracts the effects of stress chemicals. Regular practice may assist to decrease anxiety, regulate blood pressure, and increase general resistance to life's obstacles.

2. **Improved Mental Health:** Research has shown that mind-body workouts may benefit mental health by lowering symptoms of sadness, anxiety, and PTSD. These techniques help people develop mindfulness and self-awareness, allowing them to examine their thoughts and feelings without judgment. Over time, this attentive technique improves emotional control and psychological well-being.

3. **Improved Physical Health:** Mind-body exercises not only enhance the mind and emotions, but they also promote physical health. Yoga, tai chi, and other related activities use moderate movements to improve flexibility, strength, and balance. Regular involvement may help avoid injuries, relieve chronic pain, and enhance general functional mobility, especially in older persons.

4. **Stress Management:** Mind-body exercises are useful techniques for managing everyday stresses and navigating life's problems more easily. Individuals who practice mindfulness and present-moment awareness have a greater sense of clarity and perspective, allowing them to react to situations more adaptively. These techniques foster resilience and provide people with the ability to maintain homeostasis in the face of hardship.

5. **Improved Mindfulness and Presence:** Mindfulness cultivation, or consciously paying attention to the present

moment with openness and curiosity, is central to mind-body activities. Mindfulness allows people to completely connect with their experiences, cultivating a feeling of presence and aliveness. Practitioners who acquire this capacity for attentive awareness may improve their quality of life and strengthen their connection to themselves and others.

6. **Enhancement of Emotional Well-Being:** Mind-body exercises give a safe place for exploring and processing emotions. Individuals may improve their emotional resilience and self-compassion by engaging in mindful movement, breathing exercises, and meditation. These techniques help to relieve emotional strain while also promoting inner serenity and satisfaction.

7. **Cultivation of Mind-Body Awareness:** One of the primary ideas of mind-body exercises is to become aware of the body-mind relationship. Practitioners have a better grasp of how their ideas, emotions, and physical sensations are linked by engaging in mindful movement and breath awareness. This increased awareness generates a feeling of completeness and integration, which promotes overall well-being.

8. **Spiritual Connection:** Mind-body activities are often used to help people develop spiritually and realize their true selves. These activities provide a holy place for

contemplating existential concerns, connecting with a higher force, or creating an inner feeling of calm and purpose. Whether via yoga, tai chi, or meditation, people may begin on a path of self-discovery and spiritual enlightenment.

9. **Self-Care Promotion:** Participating in mind-body exercises helps to build a culture of self-care and compassion. Individuals who prioritize their well-being and devote time to nurturing their minds, bodies, and souls create a stronger feeling of self-worth and self-respect. These practices teach people to listen to their bodies, respect their needs, and live a life that promotes general health and vitality.

10. **Integration of Body, Mind, and Spirit:** Mind-body exercises are really about the integration of body, mind, and spirit, acknowledging the interdependence of all elements of human experience. Individuals who cultivate this holistic approach to health and well-being may acquire a feeling of completeness and harmony that transcends physical illnesses and mental limits. Mind-body exercises provide a doorway to comprehensive healing and self-transformation, allowing people to live with more energy, purpose, and pleasure.

To summarize, mind-body activities provide many diverse health advantages. From stress reduction and better mental health to increased physical vitality and spiritual connection, these practices provide a comprehensive approach to health and wellbeing that considers the interdependence of body, mind, and spirit. Integrating mind-body exercises into your daily routine may help you achieve a stronger feeling of balance, resilience, and vigor, improving your life on all levels.

CHAPTER 9: LIFESTYLE MODIFICATIONS

Tips For Changing Your Lifestyle To Improve Knee Health And Pain Management

Maintaining excellent knee health is critical for general mobility and quality of life, particularly as we become older. Lifestyle modifications may have a substantial impact on knee health and pain management.

1. **Maintain a Healthy Weight:** Excess weight puts additional strain on the knees, resulting in greater wear and tear. Even a small amount of weight loss may drastically lessen pressure and alleviate knee discomfort. Aim for a balanced diet rich in fruits, vegetables, whole grains, and lean meats, while limiting sugary beverages and high-fat meals.

2. **Stay Active:** Regular physical exercise promotes flexibility and strength in the muscles that support the knees. Low-impact workouts such as swimming, cycling, and walking are easy on the joints and provide significant cardiovascular benefits. Consult a healthcare physician or a physical

therapist to discover the most appropriate workouts for your situation.

3. **Strength Training:** Strengthening the muscles around the knees helps improve support and stability. Concentrate on workouts that work the quadriceps, hamstrings, and calves. Begin with low weights or resistance bands, then progressively increase as your strength grows.

4. **Proper Footwear:** Wearing supportive, well-fitting shoes may assist in preventing knee stress. Look for shoes that provide strong arch support and shock absorption. Avoid high heels, which may strain the knees and cause discomfort.

5. **Use Orthotic Devices:** Orthotic devices, such as shoe inserts or knee braces, may give extra support and relief from knee discomfort. Consult with a healthcare expert to identify the best kind of orthotic for you.

6. **Maintain Proper Posture:** Poor posture may cause knee misalignment and increase joint pressure. Maintain proper posture by standing and sitting up straight, shoulders back, and weight equally distributed on both feet.

7. **Avoid Prolonged Sitting or Standing:** To minimize stiffness and relieve strain on the knees, alternate between sitting, standing, and walking throughout the day. If you

work at a desk, try switching to a standing desk or taking regular breaks to stretch and move about.

8. **Warm-Up and Cool Down:** To lessen the chance of injury, warm up your muscles with easy stretches before starting any physical activity. After that, cool down with exercises to help relax your muscles and avoid stiffness.

9. **Stay Hydrated:** Drinking enough of water keeps your joints lubricated and minimizes the chance of inflammation. Aim to drink at least eight glasses of water every day, or more if you are active or in hot weather.

10. **Stop Smoking:** Smoking may reduce blood flow and oxygen supply to the tissues, impairing healing and increasing the risk of inflammation. Quitting smoking may improve overall health and lower your chance of knee issues.

Making these lifestyle adjustments may assist in maintaining knee health and managing discomfort. It is critical to talk with a healthcare physician before beginning any new workout or treatment plan, particularly if you already have knee problems. They may provide specialized advice and recommendations depending on your requirements and condition.

Guidelines For Maintaining A Healthy Weight, Good Eating, And Enough Water

Maintaining a healthy weight, eating properly, and staying hydrated are all important aspects of overall health, especially for seniors suffering from knee discomfort. Carrying extra weight puts additional strain on the joints, especially the knees. Each pound of body weight adds strain to the knee joints during weight-bearing movements like walking, climbing stairs, or standing up from a sitting posture. For seniors suffering from knee pain, losing weight may considerably reduce discomfort and increase mobility.

A healthy weight is normally attained by a mix of balanced eating and frequent exercise. It is critical to strive for steady, long-term weight reduction rather than fast cures or excessive diets, which may be dangerous, particularly for older persons. Consulting with a healthcare practitioner or a registered dietitian may give tailored advice on defining realistic weight reduction goals and creating an appropriate dietary plan.

In addition to weight control, specific activities that maintain muscular strength may help to support the knees and avoid additional damage. Squats, lunges, and leg presses are examples of lower-body strength training exercises that may help grow muscle mass and improve joint stability. Aerobic workouts such as walking, swimming, or cycling may help with weight loss while also improving cardiovascular health.

Proper nutrition is essential for maintaining joint health and controlling inflammation, both of which are crucial concerns for those suffering from knee discomfort. A well-balanced diet high in nutrient-dense foods may supply the critical vitamins, minerals, and antioxidants required to promote general health and lower the risk of chronic illnesses that might worsen knee pain, such as osteoarthritis.

Here are some important dietary advice for seniors with knee pain:

1. **Anti-inflammatory Foods:** Add anti-inflammatory items to your diet, such as fatty fish (salmon, mackerel), nuts and seeds (walnuts, flaxseeds), fruits (berries, cherries), vegetables (leafy greens, broccoli), and olive oil.

2. **Omega-3 Fatty Acids:** Foods high in omega-3 fatty acids, such as salmon, sardines, chia seeds, and walnuts, have been demonstrated to lower inflammation and joint discomfort.

3. **Calcium and Vitamin D:** Get enough calcium and vitamin D to maintain bone health and avoid osteoporosis, a disease that increases the risk of fractures and worsens knee pain. Dairy products, leafy greens, and fortified meals are good

sources of calcium, while vitamin D may be gained from sunshine and supplementation.

4. **Hydration:** Maintain hydration by drinking lots of water throughout the day. Proper hydration is vital for joint lubrication and may help relieve knee stiffness and soreness.

5. **Moderate Trigger Foods:** Limit your intake of items that might worsen inflammation or lead to weight gain, such as processed meals, sugary snacks and drinks, and refined carbs.

6. **Portion Control:** Use portion management to prevent overeating and maintain a healthy weight. Pay attention to your hunger and fullness signals, and pick nutrient-dense meals over empty calories.

7. **Meal Planning:** Plan nutritious meals that contain lean protein, healthy grains, fruits, and veggies. Experiment with using herbs and spices to enhance the taste of your food without using too much salt or sugar.

Proper hydration is critical for general health and well-being, including joint function and pain management. Water is essential for the health of cartilage, the cushioning tissue that cushions the joints, particularly the knees. Dehydration may cause reduced joint lubrication, increased friction, and stiffness, and worsening knee pain and discomfort.

Seniors should attempt to drink enough water throughout the day, even if they do not feel thirsty. The Institute of Medicine suggests that males drink around 3.7 liters (about 13 cups) of total water per day, while women should strive for approximately 2.7 liters (about 9 cups) of total water per day, including water from drinks and meals.

In addition to simple water, seniors may keep hydrated by eating hydrating fruits and vegetables. It is critical to manage fluid intake, particularly in hot weather or during strenuous exercise, to avoid dehydration.

In conclusion, keeping a healthy weight, a good diet, and enough hydration are critical components of controlling knee discomfort and supporting overall well-being in seniors. Seniors may improve joint health, decrease inflammation, and relieve knee pain by combining balanced eating, keeping hydrated, and obtaining or maintaining a healthy weight via lifestyle changes and frequent exercise.

Proper Footwear And Ergonomics Are Important For Preventing Knee Discomfort

Proper footwear and ergonomics are critical in decreasing knee discomfort, particularly for seniors and those with pre-existing knee difficulties. The feet and knees are inextricably linked, therefore how we support and position our feet has a direct influence on the tension and pressure on our knees.

Proper Footwear

Wearing the correct shoes is vital for preserving good alignment and decreasing knee stress. Proper footwear offers proper support, cushioning, and stability, which are critical for avoiding knee discomfort and injury.

Here are some of the main reasons why correct footwear is vital for knee health:

1. **Shock Absorption:** Walking, sprinting, and climbing stairs all cause substantial stress on the knees. Shoes with high cushioning assist absorb shock and reduce stress on the knees.

2. **Support and Stability:** Good footwear supports the arches of the feet and helps preserve good ankle alignment,

reducing stress on the knees. Shoes with proper support may assist prevent feet from overpronating (rolling inward) or supinating (rolling outward), both of which can cause knee discomfort.

3. **Alignment:** Proper knee alignment is critical to maintaining good health. Shoes that encourage good foot, ankle, and knee alignment may help lower the chance of developing or worsening knee discomfort.

4. **Comfort:** Comfortable shoes lower the risk of developing blisters, calluses, or other foot disorders that might change stride and cause knee discomfort. Shoes that fit well and are comfortable might also inspire increased physical activity, which is good for your knees.

5. **Injury Prevention:** Proper footwear may help avoid common knee injuries including sprains, strains, and fractures by providing enough support and protection during strenuous activity.

Picking the Right Shoes

When selecting shoes to decrease knee discomfort, consider the following suggestions:

- ❖ Look for shoes that provide adequate arch support and cushioning.
- ❖ Ensure that the shoes fit comfortably and allow for normal foot mobility.
- ❖ Select shoes appropriate for your activity (e.g., walking, jogging, or trekking).
- ❖ Replace worn shoes regularly to keep them supportive.

Ergonomics

In addition to appropriate footwear, ergonomics have an important role in preventing knee discomfort, particularly in the workplace. Ergonomics is the science of creating a workplace that is tailored to the worker rather than forcing the worker to conform. Proper ergonomics may assist in lessening knee strain and discomfort. *Here's why ergonomics matters for knee health:*

1. **Good Posture:** Ergonomics encourages good posture, which is critical for preserving the natural alignment of the spine, hips, and knees. Good posture lowers the likelihood of developing knee discomfort or worsening current problems.

2. **Reduced Strain:** Ergonomic workstations are intended to alleviate strain on the body, particularly the knees. Properly positioned seats, workstations, and computer displays may aid in maintaining appropriate alignment and avoiding knee discomfort.

3. **Movement:** Ergonomics promotes movement throughout the day, which is essential for minimizing stiffness and preserving joint function. Regular mobility may assist in reducing knee discomfort caused by extended sitting or standing in one posture.

4. **Equipment Adjustments:** Proper ergonomics entails changing equipment, such as seats and desks, to accommodate the individual's body size and form. This may assist in relieving tension in the knees and other joints.

Practical Pointers for Improving Ergonomics

- Use a chair with enough lumbar support and adjustable height.
- Set your computer screen at eye level to minimize straining your neck and shoulders.
- Take frequent pauses to stretch and move about.
- Use a footrest to help support your feet and relieve strain on your knees.

Proper footwear and ergonomics are critical for decreasing knee discomfort and keeping the knee healthy. Individuals who wear the correct shoes and enhance workplace ergonomics may lower their chance of developing knee discomfort, relieve current knee difficulties, and improve their overall quality of life. Investing in suitable footwear and ergonomic changes may have long-term effects on knee health and general well-being.

CHAPTER 10: LONG-TERM MAINTENANCE AND SUPPORT

Strategies For Sustaining Improvement And Avoiding Recurrence Of Knee Pain

Maintaining improvement and limiting the recurrence of knee pain is critical for seniors' mobility and quality of life. After doing knee pain reduction exercises, it is critical to practice techniques that encourage long-term joint health.

1. **Consistent Exercise Routine:** It is critical to continue with the exercise program that originally relieved knee discomfort. Walking, swimming, and cycling are all low-impact sports that help keep joints flexible and strong. Exercises that target the quadriceps, hamstrings, and calf muscles should be done regularly to help support the knee joint.

2. **Gradual Progression:** As strength and flexibility improve, progressively increase workout intensity and duration. This progressive approach lowers the danger of overuse problems and helps the body to adjust to new demands.

3. **Appropriate Form:** Maintaining appropriate form throughout workouts is critical for preventing knee discomfort from returning. Incorrect form may cause excessive stress on the joints, resulting in injury. Seniors should always seek the advice of a trained fitness instructor or physical therapist to verify that they are completing exercises appropriately.

4. **Weight Management:** Excess body weight causes extra pressure on the knees, increasing the likelihood of knee discomfort. Maintaining a healthy weight via a balanced diet and regular exercise may help lessen tension and prevent knee discomfort from recurring.

5. **Appropriate Footwear:** Wearing supportive, well-fitting shoes is essential for preserving good alignment and decreasing knee stress. Seniors should choose shoes with enough cushioning and support for their activities.

6. **Cross-Training:** Participating in a range of low-impact exercises may assist in avoiding overuse injuries and improve overall joint health. Cross-training enables seniors to alter their exercise program while reaping the advantages of regular physical activity.

7. **Warm-Up and Cool Down:** A proper warm-up before exercise and a cool-down afterward assist prepare the

muscles and joints for action while also preventing stiffness and pain. Seniors can include mild stretches into their daily routine to increase flexibility and minimize the chance of injury.

8. **Listen to Your Body:** Seniors should be aware of any indicators of discomfort or pain when exercising. Pushing through discomfort might cause more harm and should be avoided. If discomfort continues, you should alter your workouts or see a healthcare expert.

9. **Regular Health Check-ups:** Regular visits to a healthcare practitioner will assist in discovering any underlying concerns that may be causing knee discomfort. Managing disorders like arthritis and osteoporosis may help avoid future joint damage and lower the chance of recurrent knee discomfort.

10. **Include Rest Days:** Rest is an essential part of any fitness plan. Seniors should include rest days in their schedules to enable their bodies to heal and avoid overuse issues.

By adopting these measures into their everyday routines, seniors may maintain their success in controlling knee discomfort and limit the likelihood of recurrence. It's critical to approach knee health with a long-term mindset, emphasizing gradual progress and lasting behaviors.

Resources For Continued Assistance And Advice

Seniors who are experiencing knee discomfort need ongoing care and direction. Community programs and healthcare professionals play critical roles in delivering these services.

Community Programs: Community programs provide a variety of services and resources geared to the needs of seniors, including those with knee discomfort. These programs usually include:

1. **Exercise Courses:** Many community centers have specific fitness courses for elders, such as mild yoga, tai chi, and water aerobics. These programs may help you improve your flexibility, strength, and balance, all of which are essential for treating knee discomfort.

2. **Support Groups:** Support groups allow seniors to interact with others who face similar issues. Sharing experiences and coping skills may be quite helpful in managing knee discomfort and keeping a good attitude.

3. **Educational Workshops:** Workshops on nutrition, joint health, and pain management may offer seniors with useful knowledge and resources for knee discomfort.

4. **Fall Prevention Programs:** Falls are a major worry for seniors who have knee discomfort. Fall prevention programs may educate seniors on how to lower their risk of falling by including exercises, home modifications, and other safety precautions.

5. **Community Options:** Community centers often provide information on local options, such as physical therapists, orthopedic surgeons, and other healthcare experts who specialize in knee pain treatment.

Healthcare experts play an important role in controlling knee discomfort in seniors. These professions could include:

1. **Primary Care Doctors:** Primary care doctors may determine the degree of knee pain and propose suitable treatment options. They may also refer elders to experts as required.

2. **Orthopedic Specialists:** Orthopedic specialists are physicians who specialize in the treatment of musculoskeletal problems, such as knee discomfort. They may do a more thorough evaluation of knee problems and, if required, provide treatments such as physical therapy, medicines, or surgery.

3. **Physical Therapists:** Physical therapists are experts in creating exercise plans that increase mobility, relieve pain,

and prevent future damage. They may collaborate closely with elders to create a customized strategy for controlling knee discomfort.

4. **Occupational Therapists:** Occupational therapists work with elders to help them accomplish everyday tasks more comfortably and independently. They might propose home changes and assistive gadgets to lessen knee strain.

5. **Pain Management Specialists:** For seniors suffering from persistent knee pain, a pain management expert may provide a variety of pain relief options, including medicines, injections, and nerve blocks.

6. **Chiropractors and Acupuncturists:** Alternative treatments, such as chiropractic care or acupuncture, may help some seniors with knee discomfort. These practitioners may provide extra pain-management solutions.

Finally, seniors with knee discomfort have access to a range of options for continuous assistance and direction. Community programs provide a variety of services customized to elders' needs, while healthcare experts provide specialized care and treatment. Seniors may use these tools to properly manage knee discomfort and enhance their quality of life.

CONCLUSION

In this volume, we've looked at a holistic strategy for controlling knee pain in seniors using exercise and lifestyle adjustments. We've discovered that knee discomfort is a prevalent problem among seniors, typically caused by age, arthritis, or past injuries. However, with the proper counsel and resources, pain may be alleviated and quality of life improved.

Throughout this book, we've addressed the advantages of exercise for seniors with knee pain, such as increased strength, flexibility, and stability. We've tried several workouts, ranging from simple stretches to low-impact cardiovascular activities, all to relieve pain and increase mobility. We've also underlined the need for safety and good technique in avoiding future injuries.

Also, we have emphasized the importance of community programs and healthcare experts in providing continuing support and advice. Exercise courses, support groups, and educational seminars are among the activities provided by community initiatives specifically for elders. Primary care doctors, orthopedic specialists, and physical therapists play critical roles in evaluating and treating knee pain, as well as offering tailored treatment regimens.

As we get to the end of our trip, remember that controlling knee pain is an ongoing effort that demands focus and persistence. By adopting the exercises and suggestions included in this book into your daily routine, you may make proactive efforts to improve your knee health and general well-being.

Thank you for joining me on my path toward greater knee health. I hope the material and activities in this book have been beneficial to you. Remember, it's never too late to start caring for your knees, and with the appropriate attitude, you may live a more active and pain-free lifestyle.

Printed in Great Britain
by Amazon